# The Secrets of Yoga for weigh Loss

I0416067

# Copyright

Disclaimer: The information within this book is deemed correct but
as with all exercise programs due care and consideration should be
taken and it is wise to seek medical advice prior to commencing.

# Table Of Contents

## Contents

Copyright ........................................................................2

Table Of Contents ...........................................................3

Introduction ...................................................................4

How Yoga Helps With Weight Loss ..................................5

When to Practice Yoga ....................................................9

Where to Practice ..........................................................13

Eating and Drinking ......................................................15

Sun Salutation Pose ......................................................17

Double Leg Raise ..........................................................19

Corpse Pose ...................................................................20

Plough Pose ...................................................................22

Dog Pose ........................................................................23

Cobra Posture ................................................................26

Hero Pose ......................................................................27

Wheel Pose ....................................................................28

**Conclusion** ......................................................................29

**Check Out My Other Books** ........................................30

# Introduction

Yoga means union and this accurately sums up the intrinsic connection between mind, body and spirit as a result of regular practice. The average person is often under the misconception that yoga is just about stretching out the body but this is only one aspect of the benefits of yoga. Yoga is all about creating balance throughout the body, developing greater flexibility and strength as a result of performing various postures. These postures are typically held at their maximum stretch to allow the body to yield and to relax into the position but there are other types of yoga where heat and movement are required.

Yoga is non-competitive; it provides a wealth of benefits for all those who develop an interest in it and who wish to maintain a regular practice. Yoga evolves so it means that even an everyday practice routine need never stand still. The postures may not actually change but the progression will. Yoga is a gentle and safe practice and it is about letting go and embracing the changes that occur naturally. Yoga works with the mind and not against it and so it is one of the safest ways of improving health and well-being and of streamlining the body.

# How Yoga Helps With Weight Loss

Yoga may not be the exercise program that you usually associate with weight loss but with celebrity endorsements showing toned, slim physiques, it has to be said that yoga can and does help you to lose weight effectively.

Firstly, yoga with its no strain concept helps you to get in touch with your own body and it is a complete mind, body and spirit system which is effective for creating balance in your life. It gives you a chance to become more mindful, enabling you to observe what is happening to your body internally as well as to gain focus on the relationship that you have with diet and eating generally.

In fact, yoga helps you to become more flexible in your whole approach to life. So you open your mind and accept change, consider how you eat, how you stand, how you move. You can also identify and combat unhealthy and destructive patterns of eating. As you progress within yoga and you start to feel the difference that these gentle postures afford you. You start to increase the connection between your mind and body and this naturally makes you want to eat more healthily and to practice yoga more frequently, because – it feels good.

In life we learn to have unhealthy associations with food for a number of reasons. Sometimes we even block our way towards health and fitness due to our self-limitations. When you practice yoga, you start to appreciate your body and become so much more aware of how you feel, think and move. In turn, you become more comfortable in your own skin.

There are so many different types of yoga available today so you can choose the one that appeals the most. Traditionally yoga was based more on static poses and for the yoga student to feel the stretch and relax into the movement. Nowadays, there are more aerobic types of yoga available which equates to burning more calories.

People turn to yoga for many different reasons; to relax, to become more flexible and to improve certain aspects of their body. They realize that they can start to feel better about themselves and of course, to lose weight. Yoga can and does change peoples' lives for the better and there is no doubt that whichever type of yoga is chosen, providing that it is practiced regularly, your health, weight, body shape and clarity of mind is going to improve.

Consider yoga to be the transformational tool that will help you to shape up and to start feeling healthier and happier. Yoga can tighten up those less than sculpted areas, it relieves tension, increases mobility, enhances your suppleness and it can also correct any problems caused by poor posture. Yoga can tone and stretch key areas of your body and it lengthens your muscles which can help you to look longer and leaner. When you stand tall you naturally look slimmer, your body will move easier and your spine will be less rigid which in itself can make you look younger. But more than that, there are yoga poses that work on specific areas of your body such as your thyroid as this can help to balance your metabolism so that it works more efficiently. An improved metabolism means you are able to gain less weight. There are postures to improve digestion too and this can mean any sluggish or bloated feelings can ease dramatically.

Weight gain can make you feel less than healthy and it's easy to lose confidence in yourself. Yoga can help you to stop being judgmental about how you look because it creates a positive way for you to reconnect with your own body. It also enables you to master the number of jumbling thoughts that may bombard your conscious mind and if you can learn to stop thinking negatively and instead focus on all that is good about yoga, you will start to feel the difference in a matter of days.

There are styles of yoga that may be more beneficial to burning calories than others such as: Ashtanga, Bikram yoga or a Vinyasa class because the postures and breathing techniques can build heat. This can result in more calories being burned but, remember, if you are out of practice with any exercise regime it is always best to start slowly and to increase your practice as you become more used to the postures and start to feel the many benefits.

# When to Practice Yoga

When you first start practicing yoga, you will need to develop and of course maintain a regular home practice. It may not be easy when you first start out as your concentration will be on learning all of the many postures and understanding their individual benefits. It can be difficult to know what postures to practice and when and of course which postures work well together. Even those who are established with their yoga practice can be uncertain how to keep their sessions fresh and any session can be dependent on physical requirements, space at home and free time.

Part of the joy of yoga can be facing the challenges of gaining correct alignment within each pose and, it's good to join a class if possible so that you can gain some understanding of the importance of the alignment within the actual posture. But yoga must be practiced in the home environment too if you wish to see your body change shape and for all of the other incredible benefits to start.

## Planning Your Sessions

Planning ahead may seem like a chore but your yoga sessions do not have to be set in stone. Yoga is about developing an intuitive approach and this means listening to your body. Each day you should ask yourself what do you need to achieve from your yoga on that day. Maybe it is working on greater flexibility- stretching the spine and opening up the hips or if you are conscious of your weight and wish to try to lose some, your practice may need to include postures such as the shoulder stand. As you learn more about yoga, you will be able to utilize the restorative benefits and increase your energy levels or work on specific body areas incorporating the triangle perhaps so that you can streamline your waist.

To be able to choose the postures that suit you on any given day, you need to know about the principles behind any yoga sequence and if you undertake a forward bend; you must use a backward bend thereafter to ensure balance throughout the body. You may find that you are suppler in the morning and so prefer to practice the moment you climb out of bed. Stretching your body early in the morning will help to energize you and to start the day off in a positive manner. If you find you are not quite as supple during some sessions, that's ok. You may feel as if you are taking a backward step because your body feels stiff and rigid. Don't worry when this happens, because in a matter of days, you will start to feel the increased movement as progress enables your body to gain even greater stretches than you thought possible and this happens when you adjust to the movements and relax towards greater flexibility.

If you experience greater benefits practicing in the evenings, just remember that you must always practice on an empty stomach so do allow time – usually 2.5 hours after your meal. If you struggle to gain the required flexibility, never force your body, instead breathe into the posture and let your body relax into the correct position. On the out-breath, let go of any tension and you can gain extra inches of movement.

When you are planning your practice, take into account any rigid schedules you may have and try to squeeze your practice in at a time that suits. There may be some days where you cannot practice but it's important to not feel guilty, do try to practice the following day however. Regular practice is key. You don't have to practice rigidly every morning, on some days it will be far easier to practice during the evening and that's alright. Yoga is about health and well-being so it is important to go with the flow and to not stress if you cannot always practice. Even if you feel less than energetic, try to incorporate some yoga practice during the day even if it is a bout of breathing techniques or to utilize some relaxation techniques.

No doubt you will start to have your favored postures and these are usually the ones where you slip into the postures far easier than you do others. But don't limit your practice, instead, aim for a well-rounded session so that you work most of your body. Yoga works with your body on a deep level and even from day one, you will start to feel the benefits, but if you don't practice regularly, you will be missing out on your natural progression.

# Where to Practice

Ideally, when first starting to practice yoga, you should join a class so that you can learn the correct alignment of each posture ensuring that you will gain the maximum benefits of each pose. A good teacher can guide you through each extended movement and you will see and feel the difference. There are some excellent yoga classes about and if you take a look around your surrounding area, you will find one to suit in terms of style and location.

If you have some concerns about donning some traditional yoga garb because you want to tone up and lose weight, don't worry. There is some wonderful non-leotard, yoga apparel available for purchase but the only requirement really is to wear something that allows you to bend and stretch without restriction.

It's a good idea to read up on the style of choice and to visit the class prior to enrolling. Some classes let you pay per lesson but many require that you pay for the term upfront –this is to encourage students to come each week but if you are still researching your chosen style, you may not wish to do this.

Alternatively, you can purchase yoga DVD's and these come with a variety of celebrity endorsements as well as style. Some will work on the whole body, while other DVD's target those hard to tone up and exercise areas including shoulders, back and abdominals. There are also many online yoga classes that can be utilized providing you have a good Internet connection. These give you the comfort of practicing in your own home but watching a class setting and you can try out various styles and postures. Whilst it makes sense to study under a qualified teacher in the first instance, it is reassuring to know that you can at least increase your flexibility, lose weight and tone up prior to joining an established class if you so wish.

Yoga is non-competitive but you also need to feel confident and self-assured and if you do not feel 100% happy with how you look, you may find that a class is intimidating in the first instance. It's important to not let anything stand in your way from embarking on an exercise program that will improve so many areas of your life but, there are other options if joining a class does not appeal immediately.

# Eating and Drinking

Old habits can die hard and if you are looking to lose weight and to tone up, there is no alternative but to start eating healthier. Yoga can make many changes to your physical presence and can boost confidence and help you to exude a sense of contentment and well-being but it makes sense to couple this with a good nutritional plan that goes hand in hand with the physical postures.

You need to fuel your body if you wish to get the most from your yoga practice, this enables you to take a holistic approach to losing weight and looking and feeling fantastic. Eating foods that are high in nutritional values but low in toxins can only enhance your progress and this means eating lots of fruit, vegetables and whole grains.

For some yoga practitioners, food is divided into 3 categories. They are known as:

Rajasil – foods that are over processed or with too much seasoning.
Tamsik—Highly spiced, indulgent foods, may be high in sodium
Satvik- These are considered ideal and are considered as close to their origins as possible –including fresh vegetables and fruits. Understandably, Satvik foods optimize the performance of yoga as they are high in nutritional value.

There is no rule in yoga that says that you have to eat certain foods. Many yoga practitioners are vegetarians but it's more about taking a healthier approach to diet. As you start to feel and look fitter, you will naturally want to consume foods that will make you improve still further. It can be a good idea however to reduce the amount of meat that is consumed as it may contain toxins, acids, fats, cholesterol or indeed other chemicals that will not aid a yoga practice.

To follow the yoga guidance, try to eat your food while it is as fresh as possible and to savour each mouthful of food too. Make mealtimes an enjoyable time and share it with friends and family rather that rushing each mouthful.  This slowing down and appreciation of food will aid digestion and the absorption of nutrients.

# Sun Salutation Pose

The sun salutation pose is one of the most revered and dynamic of all yoga postures and the transition is slow, methodical and flowing using the breath for each transitional stage.

There are eight postures that make up the Sun Salutation Pose and they are performed in order as below:

- Mountain Pose
- Upward Salute
- Standing Forward Bend
- Lunge
- Plank Pose
- Four Limbed Staff Pose
- Upward Facing Dog Pose
- Downward Facing Dog Pose

To aid with the practice of this dynamic posture, ensure that the breathing is correct throughout. Breathe through your nose and not through your mouth.

Begin in Mountain Pose. Standing tall with your hands in prayer position at your heart level. Inhale and then stretch your arms up above you, exhaling as you lower your arms down and bend forward, chest to knee where possible. Inhale and arch your back slightly, ensuring your fingertips or flat of palms are on the floor and then extend your left leg back in a smooth movement, extending back into a lunge.
Inhale and move forward to Plank pose, lowering yourself down. Inhale, arching your body as you straighten up into Upward Dog. Exhale moving to Downward Dog. Move the left foot forward whilst inhaling and into the

lunge position. Move your right foot forward whilst exhaling and then back smoothly into an Upward Salute. Lower your arms and return to Mountain Pose.

Repeat but moving the right leg this time into the lunge poses so that you aim for balance on both sides of the body.

Repeat as required.

The key to performing this sequence of postures well is to practice each pose within carefully and once you know the poses and then the sequence, mindfully work through them utilizing the breath as you do so.
Benefits:

The Sun Salutation sequence when done at a good pace (mindfully) is a wonderful way to lose weight but do not forego accuracy for speed. It increases the cardiovascular work-out but actually tones and stretches muscles throughout the body. Importantly, the Sun Salutation pose helps to maintain your good health, whilst improving your digestive system, the respiratory and circulatory system.

# Double Leg Raise

One of the key areas which people want to tone up is often the midriff and in fact, core muscles are the most important but difficult areas to keep in optimal condition. Yoga generally can help to keep your body flexible and toned but the Double Leg Raise pose can help to tighten up your abdominals and you should try to incorporate this into your yoga practice most days.

Lie flat on the floor, body relaxed and focus your gaze on the ceiling. Inhale deeply and raise both legs –keeping them straight. Keep your buttocks on the floor

Exhale and lower both legs to the floor – using the abdominal muscles, trying to keep the movement slow and flowing.

Repeat as many times as required. As you gain control over this movement, try to keep your feet off the floor in their extended position and this will increase the workout for your abdominals.

Benefits

Double Leg Raises work your abdominals, waist, hips and back as well as stretching all of the leg muscles.

# Corpse Pose

The corpse posture usually occurs at the end of any yoga session although can be used in between to determine how your body feels after a deep yoga sequence. It is important to feel comfortable within this posture so that you can learn to anticipate how your body is feeling and to eradicate any tension. It is the position that you assume when you wish to enter deep relaxation.

Lie flat on the floor, ensuring that you can feel the floor against the length of your spine. To be sure you are in the correct alignment, lift your pelvis off of the floor and then relax back, and lie comfortably.
Extend the base of your skull away from the neck allowing space in the neckline.
If you feel uncomfortable or unsure that you are in the correct position, move your body from side to side in a rocking motion. Reach your arms up towards the ceiling and over your head and then back down to your sides, allowing space from your torso to your hands. Turn your arms outwards and palms upwards.

Visualise the tension leaving your body from the tips of your toes up through to your skull. Many people retain tension in their faces so make a conscious effort to soften your face, letting your eyes sink back into your head and ensure you are not clenching your jaw.

Stay in this pose for five to ten minutes and enjoy the feeling of peace within your body after your yoga practice. Try to turn your attention inward and to not let the mind wander.

To finish, exhale and roll to the side, lifting your body as your hands push against the floor. Your head should be the last to come up.

Benefits:

- Calms the mind.
- Relieves stress
- Eases and reduces fatigue and headaches.
- Lowers blood pressure
- Helps to relieve mild cases of depression
- Helps to improve deep sleep

# Plough Pose

From the Shoulder Stand pose, exhale and bend your body from the hips and slowly lower your toes to the floor over and beyond your head. Keep your legs straight, extended and the movement controlled.

Ensure correct positioning once your toes are on the floor by lifting the top of your thighs and your tailbone so that they lift towards the ceiling. Soften your throat and try to create space between the chin and the sternum.

Keep your hands on your back and continue to push up towards the ceiling. If you are comfortable, you can release your hands and stretch them out on the floor opposing your legs. Hold the pose for 1-5 minutes but do not strain. To come out of the pose, place your hands onto your back and return to the Shoulder Stand on an exhalation. Then roll down until you are in the corpse position and take time to settle your body and remove tension from your neck and spine.

Benefits:

- Stimulates the thyroid gland
- Stretches out the shoulders and spine
- Relieves symptoms of the menopause
- Releases feelings of stress and fatigue
- Eases backache
- Can improve insomnia and headaches
- Quietens the brain

# Dog Pose

Downward Facing Dog

Benefits:

- Stretches calves, foot arches, hamstrings and hands
- Strengthens arms and shoulders
- Strengthens your back
- Improves digestion
- Elongates your spine
- Helps to release tension from your spine
- Eases menopausal symptoms
- Calms the nervous system and alleviates feelings of stress

On your hands and knees, place your palms just forward from your shoulders. Your index finger should be forwards, fingers spread and your knees should be under your hips for correct alignment. With your toes tucked underneath, inhale and lift your knees from the floor and push your bottom up towards the ceiling.

Initially, your knees should be slightly bent and heels off of the floor. Elongate your spine and try to imagine your abdomen moving towards your heels. Lengthen your legs and lower your heels slowly mindful of any slight feelings of strain.

Roll your heels outwards just slightly and push down in this position while imagining your upper things rolling inward slightly.

Try to widen your shoulder blades and keep your neck long. Your head should be in alignment with your arms.

Do not lock your knee joints or elbows.

Try to keep your weight evenly distributed through hands and feet.

Hold for several breaths and then release moving back into child's pose to rest or onto the next posture.

## Upward Facing Dog Pose

Lie on the floor face down. Place the tops of your feet on the floor and imagine your legs stretching back. Now, bend your elbows so that you are leaning on your forearms. Spread your palms. On an in-breath, press your hands against the floor and straighten your arms lifting your torso off of the floor as you do so. You will find that you can lift the hips and upper thighs from the floor too. Push your tailbone towards your pubis and imagine your pubis lifting towards your navel area. Do not tense your buttocks, just keep them firm.

Look straight ahead or you can also tip your head back just slightly. Do not tighten the throat or compress your neck. Relax back onto the floor after 15-30 seconds with an exhalation and breathe normally.

Note: This is one of the Sun Salutation postures but it can be practiced alone.

Benefits:

- Strengthens shoulders, arms and wrists
- Strengthens chest and lungs.
- Aids asthma
- Strengthens the abdomen
- Helps to firm the buttocks
- Improves overall posture
- Helps to release stress or ease mild depression
- Stimulates inner abdominal organs

# Cobra Posture

The Cobra posture has many benefits:

- It decreases stiffness and tension in the lower back and strengthens the spine
- It can ease symptoms associated with sciatica
- It strengthens your arms and shoulders
- It can improve any irregularities with the menstrual cycle
- It can firm and tone your buttocks
- It improves circulation and digestion
- It relieves fatigue and also feelings of stress
- It can improve mood
- It stimulates those inner organs

Lie face down on the floor, arms by your side. Place your hands on the floor directly under your shoulders and ensure that your elbows are next to your body. Press your feet and thighs firmly against the floor.

Inhale and straighten your arms, lifting your chest up off the floor. Resist the urge to clench your buttocks and keep the connection from your pubis to the floor. This will prevent you from lifting your hips off the floor.

Hold this pose for as long as is comfortable but up to 30 seconds before releasing the extreme pose and lying back down on the floor. Take your hands to the side of your body and rest your face on one side, breathe deeply and then repeat the movement.

Tip: Do not overdo the stretch. Keep your hips on the floor and extend through the spine.

# Hero Pose

The hero pose may look simple but it has a great many benefits including:

It is therapeutic for asthma
It aids high blood pressure.
It improves gas and aids digestion
Strengthens knees, ankles and thighs
Strengthens the arches
Can alleviate menopausal symptoms
Can reduce swelling of the legs as a result of pregnancy

Kneel on the floor, placing a folded blanket underneath your knees and feet if required. Ensure that your inner knees are together and then slide your feet apart and then sit down in between your feet; the tops of your feet should be flat on the floor. Exhale and sit back.

You may find it difficult to sit comfortably with your buttocks flat on the floor as it can put pressure onto the knee joints and in this case, place a book or yoga block between your feet. Sit evenly. Turn your thighs inwards and lay your hands on top of your thighs. Remain conscious of your posture.

Remain in the posture for approximately 30 seconds initially and increase for up to 1 minute. Eventually, stay within the pose for up to 5 minutes. Come out of the posture carefully by lifting your buttocks up off of the floor and sit to one side, easing your legs out from underneath you.

# Wheel Pose

Wheel pose may seem a daunting posture if you are not supple but once you have increased the flexibility to your spine, it's a beautiful pose to try and offers many benefits including:

- It lengthens and strengthens the vertebrae. It creates space within the spine and keeps it healthy avoiding the loss of inches later in life.

- It strengthens your abdomen, legs, arms and wrists. It also strengthens the shoulders.

- Regular practice of this powerful posture will serve to open up the chest area, increasing oxygen intake and improving respiration. This is an excellent posture for sufferers of asthma.

- The wheel pose can also help to balance hormones and to enhance your nervous system.

- The wheel pose is excellent for trimming fat from your stomach area.

- It increases the flexibility of the hips

- It counteracts feelings of stress, anxiety and depression and boosts energy on a physical and mental level.

- It stimulates the thyroid and pituitary glands.

- 

Instructions:

Lie on your back. Bend your knees and bring your feet parallel close to your buttocks. Bend your elbows, bringing your hands under your shoulders, palms facing downwards. Fingertips should be pointing towards your feet. Inhale and lift your hips off of the floor, pressing your palms down into the floor as you do so.

Place the crown of your head onto the floor and pause. Check that your elbows are parallel. Then straighten your arms lifting the head off the floor. Keep your legs parallel and imagine that you are reaching up aiming your chest towards a wall. Straighten your legs and hold for up to three minutes. This is a very strong pose so start slowly and hold only for a few seconds initially and then increase.

To come down, simply tuck your chin towards your chest and then lower yourself down slowly. Rest prone on the floor and allow any tension to dissipate.

Tip: Be careful if you have any heart irregularities, high or low blood pressure or back injuries.

# Conclusion

Thank you again for downloading this book!
Finally, if you enjoyed this book, please take the time to share your thoughts and post a review on Amazon. It'd be greatly appreciated!

Thank you and good luck!

# Check Out My Other Books

Below you'll find some of my other popular books that are popular on Amazon and Kindle as well. Simply click on the links below to check them out. Alternatively, you can visit my author page on Amazon to see other work done by me.

**http://www.amazon.com/NrBooks/e/B00ET2BG9Y/**

If the links do not work, for whatever reason, you can simply search for these titles on the Amazon website to find them.

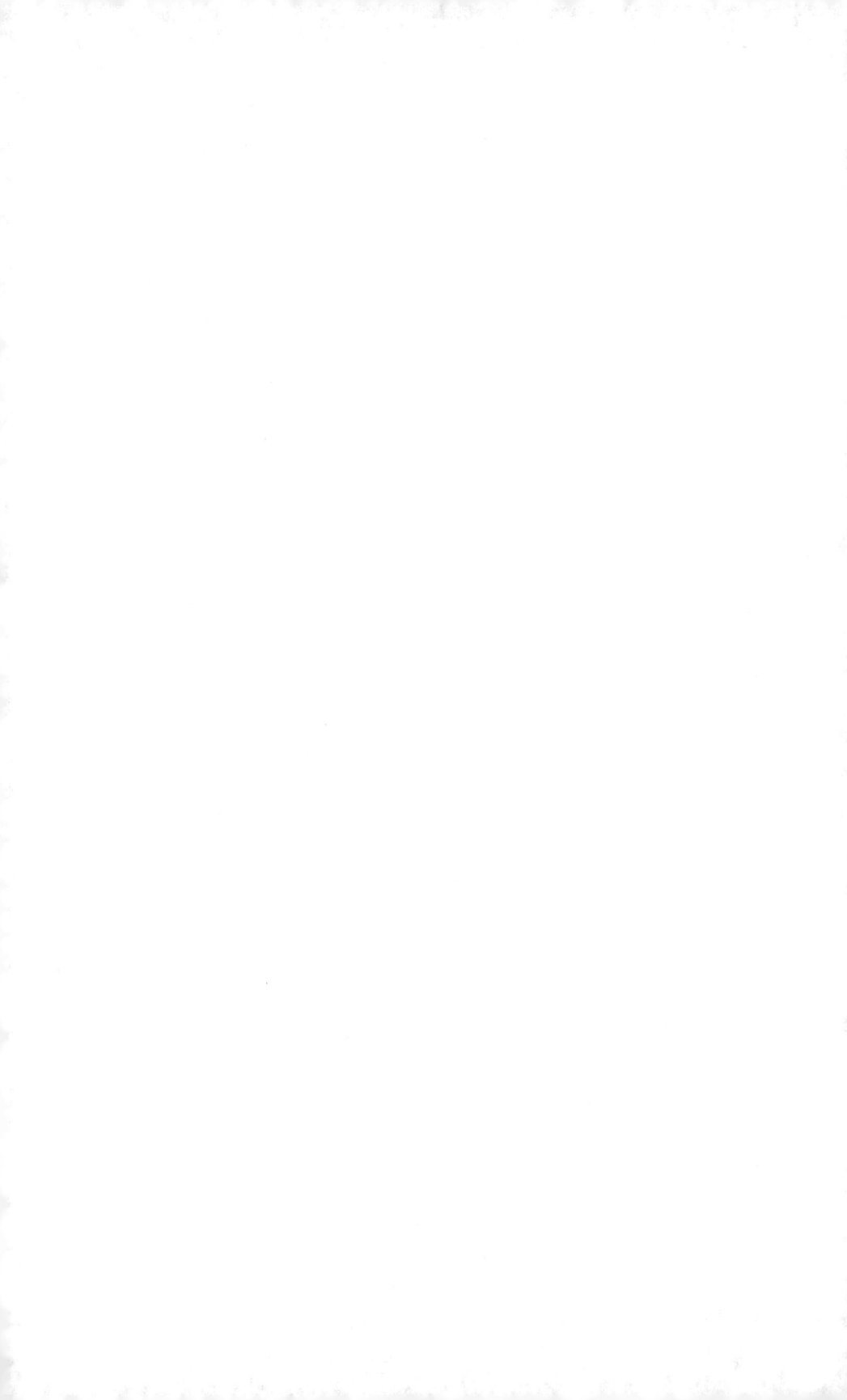

www.ingramcontent.com/pod-product-compliance
Lightning Source LLC
Chambersburg PA
CBHW070940290526
45795CB00003B/1093